The Best   Pressure Cooker Meat Recipes for Moms

Quick and Easy Poultry Recipes

Robin E. Clayton

Sommario

Introduction

The Ninja Foodi multi-cooker is one of the appliances that everybody need to have in their kitchen. The tool can replace four small tools: slow-moving cooker, air fryer, pressure cooker and also dehydrator.

This recipe book contains some of the dishes we have attempted with the multi-cooker. The dishes vary from morning meal, side meals, poultry, pork, soups, seafood, desserts, as well as pasta. Furthermore, we've put together lots of vegetarian recipes you ought to try. We produced these dishes considering novices which's why the cooking treatment is methodical. Besides, the recipes are scrumptious, appreciate analysis.

Meet

Sticky St. Louis Ribs

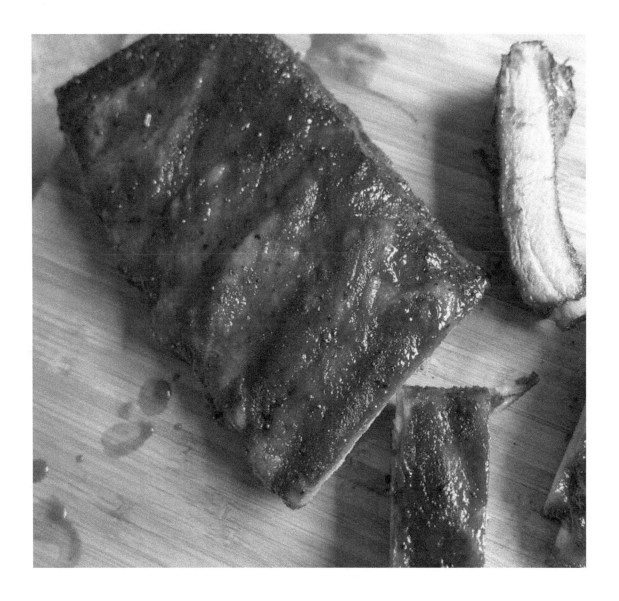

INGREDIENTS (4 Servings)

1/4 cup of barbecue spice rub

2 tablespoons of brown sugar

2 tablespoons of kosher salt

1 rack of uncooked St. Louis ribs (3 to three 1/2 lb)

1/2 cup of beer

1 cup of barbecue sauce

DIRECTIONS (PREP + COOK TIME: 51 MINUTES) Cut the ribs into three and add them to a bowl. Add the spice rub, brown sugar, and salt. Stir. Pour the beer into the Foodi pot and put your seasoned ribs into the basket. Fix the basket in the pot and close the pressure lid. Cook your ribs on high mode for 20 minutes. Quick release the pressure and open the lid. Close the crisping lid reset the Ninja unit to air crisp mode. Set the cooking temperatures to 400°F and time to 15 minutes. Open the lid after 10minutes and brush the rib mixture with the BBQ sauce. Resume cooking. Cooking ends when the internal temperature drops to 185°F. Serve!

Asian Baby Ribs

INGREDIENTS (4 Servings)

2 tablespoons sesame oil

1 tablespoon cayenne pepper

½ cup soy sauce

2 tablespoons rice vinegar

1 small onion, minced

8 garlic cloves, minced

1 tablespoon grated fresh ginger

1 (3-pound) rack baby back ribs, cut into quarters

½ cup water

¼ cup honey

Sesame seeds

DIRECTIONS (Prep + Cook Time: 30-35 minutes) In a mixing bowl, combine the soy sauce, rice vinegar, sesame oil, cayenne pepper, garlic, ginger, and onion.   In another bowl, add the ribs and add the mixture over, cover, and refrigerate for 30 minutes.   Take Ninja Foodi multi-cooker, arrange it over a cooking platform, and open the top lid.   In the pot, arrange a reversible rack and place the Crisping Basket over the rack. In the basket, add the ribs and set aside the marinade in another bowl.   Seal the multi-cooker by locking it with the pressure lid; ensure to keep the pressure release valve locked/sealed.   Select "PRESSURE" mode and select the "HI" pressure level. Then, set timer to 10 minutes and press "STOP/START"; it will start the cooking process by building up inside pressure.   When the timer goes off, quickly release pressure by adjusting the pressure valve to the VENT. After pressure gets released, open the pressure lid. Add the reserved marinade over the ribs.   Seal the multi-cooker by locking it with the crisping lid; ensure to keep the pressure release valve locked/sealed.   Select the "AIR CRISP" mode and adjust the 400°F temperature level. Then, set timer to 15 minutes and press "STOP/START"; it will start the cooking process by building up inside pressure. After 10 minutes, open the lid and brush the ribs with the honey.   When the timer goes off, quickly release pressure by adjusting the pressure valve to the VENT. After pressure gets released, open the Crisping Lid. Slice the ribs and serve warm with the sesame seeds on top.

Jamaican Bean Pork

INGREDIENTS (4 Servings)

1 habanero chile, seeded and minced

2 tablespoons packed brown sugar

2 tablespoons sherry vinegar

2 garlic cloves, minced

2 tablespoons grated peeled ginger

2 ½ pounds boneless country ribs

1 teaspoon kosher salt

¼ cup chicken stock

½ teaspoon ground cinnamon

2 teaspoons ground allspice

1 teaspoon dried thyme leaves

1 (15-ounce) can kidney beans, drained and rinsed

2 cups cooked rice

DIRECTIONS (Prep + Cook Time: 40-45 minutes) Sprinkle the ribs with the salt. Take Ninja Foodi multi-cooker, arrange it over a cooking platform, and open the top lid.   In the pot, add the stock. Add the habanero, garlic, ginger, brown sugar, vinegar, allspice, thyme, and cinnamon. Stir to combine.   Seal the multi-cooker by locking it with the pressure lid; ensure to keep the pressure release valve locked/sealed.   Select "PRESSURE" mode and select the "HI" pressure level. Then, set timer to 25 minutes and press "STOP/START"; it will start the cooking process by building up inside pressure.   When the timer goes off, quickly release pressure by adjusting the pressure valve to the VENT. After pressure gets released, open the pressure lid. Take out the ribs and in the pot, mix in the beans and rice.   Place a reversible rack inside the pot. Place the ribs over the rack.   Seal the multi-cooker by locking it with the Crisping Lid; ensure to keep the pressure release valve locked/sealed.   Select "BROIL" mode and select the "HI" pressure level. Then, set timer to 10 minutes and press "STOP/START"; it will start the cooking process by building up inside pressure. After 5 minutes, turn the ribs.   When the timer goes off, quickly release pressure by adjusting the pressure valve to the VENT. After pressure gets released, open the Crisping Lid. Serve warm.

Pork Green Apple

INGREDIENTS (4 Servings)

3/4 cup red wine

4 garlic cloves, minced

1 ½ pound pork tenderloin, cubed

2 green apple, cored and cut into wedges

2 tablespoons butter, melted

Black pepper (finely ground) and salt to the taste

DIRECTIONS (Prep + Cook Time: 40-45 minutes) Take a baking pan; grease it with some cooking spray, vegetable oil, or butter. Add all the ingredients and combine them. Take Ninja Foodi multi-cooker, arrange it over a cooking platform, and open the top lid. In the pot, add water and place a reversible rack inside the pot. Place the pan over the rack. Seal the multi-cooker by locking it with the Crisping Lid; ensure to keep the pressure release valve locked/sealed. Select "BAKE/ROAST" mode and adjust the 360°F temperature level. Then, set timer to 35 minutes and press "STOP/START"; it will start the cooking process by building up inside pressure. When the timer goes off, quickly release pressure by adjusting the pressure valve to the VENT. After pressure gets released, open the Crisping Lid. Serve warm.

Drunken Lamb Potato

INGREDIENTS (4 Servings)

2 tablespoons canola oil

2 Yukon gold potatoes, cut into 1-inch pieces

2 carrots, cut into 2-inch pieces

2 bone-in lamb shanks, 2 to 2 ½ pounds each

Kosher salt

Black pepper (ground)

2 parsnips, peeled and cut into 2-inch pieces

1 (14-ounce) bag pearl onions

1 bottle red wine of 750 ml

1 tablespoon chopped fresh rosemary

1 cup chicken stock

DIRECTIONS (Prep + Cook Time: 20-25 minutes)

Season the lamb shanks with salt and black pepper. Take Ninja Foodi multi-cooker, arrange it over a cooking platform, and open the top lid.   In the pot, add the oil, Select "SEAR/SAUTÉ" mode and select "MD: HI" pressure level. Press "STOP/START." After about 4-5 minutes, the oil will start simmering.   Add the lamb and stir-cook for about 8-10 minutes to brown evenly. Set aside.   Add the potatoes, carrots, parsnips, and pearl onions, stir-cook for 5 minutes. Mix the red wine, chicken stock, and rosemary. Add the lamb shanks and stir gently.   Seal the multi-cooker by locking it with the pressure lid, ensure to keep the pressure release valve locked/sealed.   Select the "SLOW COOK" mode and select the "HI" pressure level. Then after, set timer to 4 hours minutes and press "STOP/START," it will start the cooking process by building up inside pressure.   When the timer goes off, quickly release pressure by adjusting the pressure valve to the VENT. After pressure gets released, open the pressure lid.   Serve warm.

Steak Pineapple Delight

INGREDIENTS (4 Servings)

½ medium pineapple, cored and diced

1 jalapeno, seeded and stemmed, diced

1 medium red onion, diced

4 pieces filet mignon steaks, 6-8 ounces each

1 tablespoon canola oil

Salt and pepper to taste

1 tablespoon lime juice

¼ cup cilantro leaves, chopped

Chili powder and ground coriander

DIRECTIONS (Prep + Cook Time: 13-18 minutes)

Rub fillets with oil evenly, season them well with salt and pepper Pre-heat Ninja Foodi by pressing the "GRILL" option and setting it to "HIGH" and timer to 8 minutes Let it pre-heat until you hear a beep Arrange fillets over grill grate, lock lid and cook for 4 minutes until the internal temperature reaches 125 degrees F Take a mixing bowl and add pineapple, onion, jalapeno, mix well Add lime juice, cilantro, chili powder, coriander and combine Serve fillets with the pineapple mixture on top Enjoy!

Coca-Cola Beef Roast

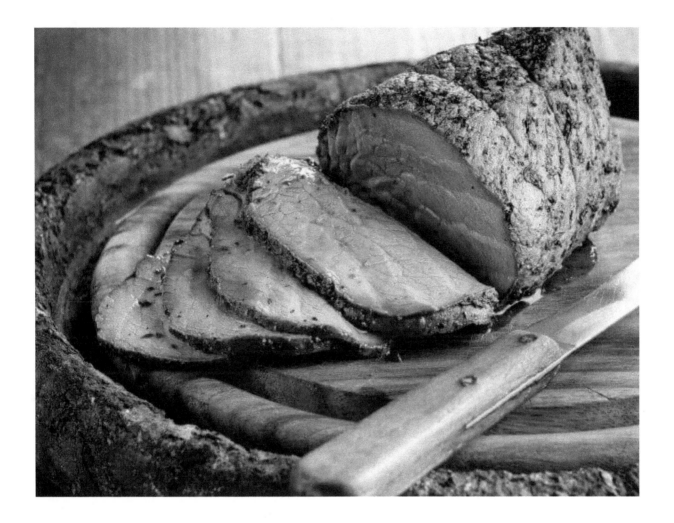

INGREDIENTS (4 Servings)

2 pounds beef sirloin roast

2 garlic cloves, minced

1 can cola

½ cup of water

1 teaspoon salt

1 teaspoon pepper

1 bay leaf

DIRECTIONS (Prep + Cook Time: 45-50 minutes)

Pre-heat Ninja Foodi by pressing the "ROAST" option and setting it to "400 Degrees F" and timer to 40 minutes Let it pre-heat until you hear a beep Arrange the listed ingredients in Grill Basket Lock lid and cook until the timer goes to zero Serve and enjoy!

Mushroom Soy Beef

INGREDIENTS (2 Servings)

8 ounces shiitake mushrooms, sliced

2 tablespoon dark soy sauce

1 teaspoon olive oil

1 pound beef meat, cut into strips

1 yellow onion, chopped

Black pepper (ground) and salt to taste

DIRECTIONS (Prep + Cook Time: 17-22 minutes)

Take Ninja Foodi multi-cooker, arrange it over a cooking platform, and open the top lid.   In the pot, add the oil, Select "SEAR/SAUTÉ" mode and select "MD: HI" pressure level. Press "STOP/START." After about 4-5 minutes, the oil will start simmering.   Add the onions and cook (while stirring) until they become softened and translucent for 3-4 minutes. Add the mushrooms, soy sauce, and beef, stir-cook for another 2-3 minutes. Season with salt and black pepper. Seal the multi-cooker by locking it with the pressure lid, ensure to keep the pressure release valve locked/sealed. Select "PRESSURE" mode and select the "HI" pressure level. Then after, set timer to 8 minutes and press "STOP/START," it will start the cooking process by building up inside pressure. When the timer goes off, naturally release inside pressure for about 8-10 minutes. Then, quick-release pressure by adjusting the pressure valve to the VENT. Serve warm.

Adobo Cubed Steak

INGREDIENTS (4 Servings)

8 steaks, cubed, 28 ounces pack Pepper to taste

1 and ¾ teaspoons adobo seasoning

1 can (8 ounces) tomato sauce

1/3 cup green pitted olives

2 tablespoons brine

1 small red pepper

½ a medium onion, sliced

DIRECTIONS (PREP + COOK TIME: 30 MINUTES)

Chop peppers, onions into ¼ inch strips Prepare beef by seasoning with adobo and pepper . Add into Ninja Foodi Add remaining ingredients and Lock lid, cook on HIGH pressure for 25 minutes Release pressure naturally. Serve and enjoy!

A Keto-Friendly Philly Willy Steak And Cheese

INGREDIENTS (4 Servings)

2 tablespoons olive oil

2 large onion, sliced

8 ounces mushrooms, sliced 1-2 teaspoons

Keto friendly steak seasoning

1 tablespoon butter

2 pounds beef chuck roast

12 cup beef stock

DIRECTIONS (PREP + COOK TIME: 50 MINUTES)

Set your Ninja Foodi to Saute mode and add oil, let it heat up Rub seasoning over roast and Saute for 1-2 minutes per side Remove and add butter, onion. Add mushrooms, pepper, stock, and roast Lock lid and cook on HIGH pressure for 35 minutes. Naturally, release pressure over 10 minutes Shred meat and sprinkle cheese if using, enjoy!

Beef Stew

INGREDIENTS (20 Servings)

1 pound beef roast

4 cups beef broth

3 garlic cloves, chopped

1 carrot, chopped

2 celery stalks, chopped

2 tomatoes, chopped

½ white onion, chopped

¼ teaspoon salt

1/8 teaspoon ground black pepper

DIRECTIONS (PREP + COOK TIME: 20 MINUTES)

Add listed ingredients to your Ninja Foodi and lock lid, cook on HIGH pressure for 10 minutes Quick release pressure. Open the lid and shred the bee using forks, serve and enjoy!

Juiciest Keto Bacon Strips

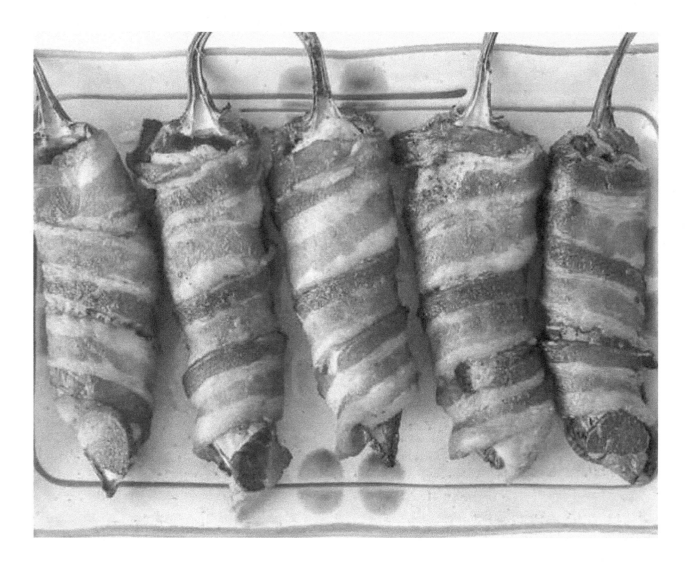

INGREDIENTS (2 Servings)

10 bacon strips

¼ teaspoon chili flakes

1/3 teaspoon salt

¼ teaspoon basil, dried

DIRECTIONS (PREP + COOK TIME: 12 MINUTES)

Rub the bacon strips with chili flakes, dried basil, and salt Turn on your air fryer and place the bacon on the rack Lower the air fryer lid. Cook the bacon at 400F for 5 minutes Cook for 3 minutes more if the bacon is not fully cooked. Serve and enjoy!

Quick Picadillo Dish

INGREDIENTS (4 Servings)

½ pound lean ground beef

2 garlic cloves, minced

½ large onion, chopped

1 teaspoon salt

1 tomato, chopped

½ red bell pepper, chopped

1 tablespoon cilantro

½ can (4 ounces) tomato sauce

1 teaspoon ground cumin

1-2 bay leaves

2 tablespoons green olives, capers

2 tablespoons brine

3 tablespoons water

DIRECTIONS (PREP + COOK TIME: 30 MINUTES)

Set your Ninja Foodi to Saute mode and add meat, salt, and pepper, slightly brown Add garlic, tomato, onion, cilantro and Saute for 1 minute Add olives, brine, leaf, cumin, and mix. Pour in sauce, water, and stir Lock lid and cook on HIGH pressure for 15 minutes. Quick release pressure

Generous Shepherd's Pie

INGREDIENTS (4 Servings)

2 cups of water

4 tablespoons butter

4 ounces cream cheese

1 cup mozzarella

1 whole egg

Salt and pepper to taste

1 tablespoon garlic powder

2-3 pounds ground beef

1 cup frozen carrots

8 ounces mushrooms, sliced

1 cup beef broth

DIRECTIONS (PREP + COOK TIME: 25 MINUTES)

Add water to Ninja Foodi, arrange cauliflower on top, lock lid and cook for 5 minutes on HIGH pressure Quick release and transfer to a blender, add cream cheese, butter, mozzarella cheese, egg, pepper, and salt. Blend well. Drain water from Ninja Foodi and add beef Add carrots, garlic powder, broth and pepper, and salt Add in cauliflower mix and lock lid, cook for 10 minutes on HIGH pressure Release pressure naturally over 10 minutes. Serve and enjoy!

Hybrid Beef Prime Roast

INGREDIENTS (4 Servings)

2 pounds chuck roast

1 tablespoon olive oil

1 teaspoon salt

1 teaspoon ground black pepper

1 teaspoon onion powder

1 teaspoon garlic powder

4 cups beef stock

DIRECTIONS (PREP + COOK TIME: 55 MINUTES)

Place roast in Ninja Food pot and season it well with salt and pepper Add oil and set the pot to Saute mode, sear each side of roast for 3 minutes until slightly browned . Add beef broth, onion powder, garlic powder, and stir Lock lid and cook on HIGH pressure for 40 minutes Once the timer goes off, naturally release pressure over 10 minutes Open the lid and serve hot. Enjoy!

Hearty Korean Ribs

INGREDIENTS (6 Servings)

1 teaspoon olive oil

2 green onions, cut into

1-inch length

3 garlic cloves, smashed

3 quarter sized ginger slices

4 pounds beef short ribs,

3 inches thick, cut into

3 rib portions

½ cup of water

½ cup coconut aminos

¼ cup dry white wine

2 teaspoons sesame oil

Mince green onions for serving

DIRECTIONS (PREP + COOK TIME: 55 MINUTES)

Set your Ninja Foodi to "SAUTE" mode and add oil, let it shimmer Add green onions, garlic, ginger, Saute for 1 minute Add short ribs, water, amines, wine, sesame oil, and stir until the ribs are coated well Lock lid and cook on HIGH pressure for 45 minutes . Release pressure naturally over 10 minutes Remove short ribs from pot and serve with the cooking liquid. Enjoy!

Beef And Broccoli Platter

INGREDIENTS (4 Servings)

3 pounds beef chuck roast, cut into thin strips

1 tablespoon olive oil

1 yellow onion, peeled and chopped

½ cup beef stock

1 pound broccoli florets

2 teaspoons toasted sesame oil

2 tablespoons arrowroot For Marinade

1 cup coconut aminos

1 tablespoon sesame oil

2 tablespoons fish sauce

5 garlic cloves, peeled and minced

3 red peppers, dried and crushed

½ teaspoon Chinese five spice powder

Toasted sesame seeds, for serving

DIRECTIONS (PREP + COOK TIME: 30 MINUTES)

Take a bowl and mix in coconut aminos, fish sauce, 1 tablespoon sesame oil, garlic, five spice powder, crushed red pepper and stir Add beef strips to the bowl and toss to coat. Keep it on the side for 10 minutes Set your Ninja Foodi to "Saute" mode and add oil, let it heat up, add onion and stir cook for 4 minutes. Add beef and marinade, stir cook for 2 minutes. Add stock and stir Lock the pressure lid of Ninja Foodi and cook on HIGH pressure for 5 minutes Release pressure naturally over 10 minutes Mix arrowroot with ¼ cup liquid from the pot and gently pour the mixture back to the pot and stir Place a steamer basket in the pot and add broccoli to the steamer rack, lock lid and cook on HIGH pressure for 3 minutes more, quick release pressure Divide the dish between plates and serve with broccoli, toasted sesame seeds and enjoy!

Marked Beef Goulash

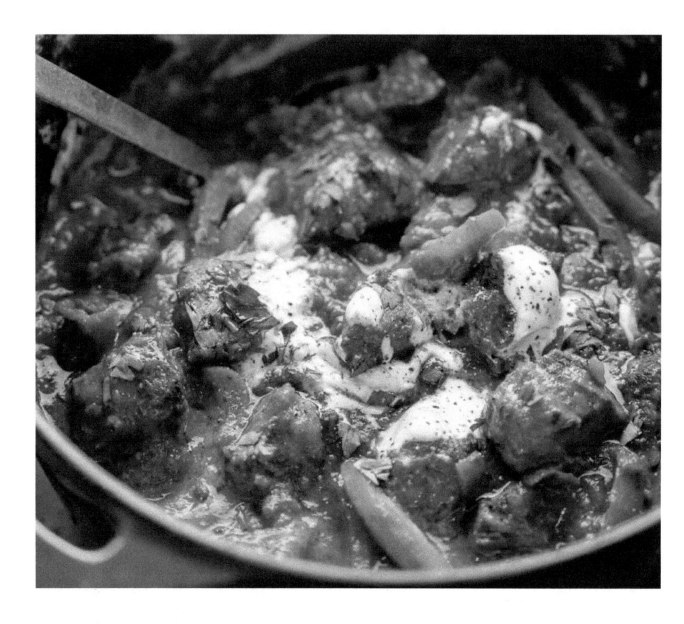

INGREDIENTS (4 Servings)

1-2 pounds extra lean beef, ground

2 teaspoons olive oil + 11 teaspoons extra

1 large red bell pepper, stemmed and seeded

1 large onion, cut into short strips

1 tablespoon garlic, minced

2 tablespoons sweet paprika

½ teaspoon hot paprika

4 cups beef stock

2 cans tomatoes, diced and petite

DIRECTIONS (PREP + COOK TIME: 30 MINUTES)

Set your Ninja Foodi to Saute mode and add 2 teaspoons of olive oil Add ground beef to the pot and cook, making sure to stir it until it breaks apart Once the beef is browned, transfer it to a bowl. Cut the steam off the pepper and deseed them and cut into strips. Cut the onion into short strips as well Add a teaspoon of olive oil to the pot alongside pepper and onion Saute for 3-4 minutes.Add minced garlic, sweet paprika, hot paprika and cook for 2-3 minutes Add beef stock alongside the tomatoes. Add ground beef Allow it to cook for about 15 minutes on Soup mode over the low pressure Once done, quick release the pressure and have fun!

Meat Dredged Loaf

INGREDIENTS (6 Servings)

½ cup onion, chopped

2 garlic cloves, minced

¼ cup sugar-free ketchup

1 pound grass fed lean ground beef

½ cup green bell pepper, seeded and chopped

1 cup cheddar cheese, grated

2 organic eggs, beaten

1 teaspoon dried thyme, crushed

3 cups fresh spinach, chopped

6 cups mozzarella cheese, freshly grated

Black pepper to taste

DIRECTIONS (PREP + COOK TIME: (1 hours and 20 MINUTES)

Take a bowl and add all of the listed ingredients except cheese and spinach Place a wax paper on a smooth surface and arrange the meat over it Top with spinach, cheese and roll the paper around the paper to form a nice meatloaf Remove wax paper and transfer loaf to your Ninja Foodi Lock lid and select "Bake/Roast" mode, setting the timer to 70 minutes and temperature to 380 degrees F. Let it bake and take the dish out once done. Serve and enjoy!

Spiritual Indian Beef Dish

INGREDIENTS (4 Servings)

½ yellow onion, chopped

1 tablespoon olive oil

2 garlic cloves, minced

1 jalapeno pepper, chopped

1 cup cherry tomatoes, quartered

1 teaspoon fresh lemon juice

1-2 pounds grass-fed ground beef

1-2 pounds fresh collard greens, trimmed and chopped Spices

1 teaspoon cumin, ground

½ teaspoon ginger, ground

1 teaspoon coriander, ground

½ teaspoon fennel seeds, ground

½ teaspoon cinnamon, ground

Salt and pepper to taste

½ teaspoon turmeric, ground

DIRECTIONS (PREP + COOK TIME: 35 MINUTES)

Set your Ninja Foodi to sauté mode and add garlic, onions sauté for 3 minutes. Add jalapeno pepper, beef, and spices Lock lid and cook on Medium-HIGH pressure for 15 minutes Release pressure naturally over 10 minutes, open lid Add tomatoes, collard greens and sauté for 3 minutes Stir in lemon juice, salt, and pepper. Stir well Once the dish is ready, transfer the dish to your serving bowl and enjoy!

All-Tim Favorite Beef Chili

INGREDIENTS (4 Servings)

1 and ½ pounds ground beef

1 sweet onion, peeled and chopped

Salt and pepper to taste

28 ounces canned tomatoes, diced

17 ounces beef stock

6 garlic clove, peeled and chopped

7 jalapeno peppers, diced

2 tablespoons olive oil

4 carrots, peeled and chopped

3 tablespoons chili powder

1 bay leaf

1 teaspoon chili powder

DIRECTIONS (PREP + COOK TIME: 50 MINUTES)

Set your Ninja Foodi to "Saute" mode and add half of the oil, let it heat up Add beef and stir brown for 8 minutes, transfer to a bowl Add remaining oil to the pot and let it heat up, add carrots, onion, jalapenos, garlic and stir Saute for 4 minutes. Add tomatoes and stir Add bay leaf, stock, chili powder, chili powder, salt, pepper, and beef, stir and lock lid Cook on HIGH pressure for 25 minutes . Release pressure naturally over 10 minutes Stir the chili and serve. Enjoy!

Sesame Beef Ribs

INGREDIENTS (6 Servings)

1 tablespoon sesame oil

2 garlic cloves, peeled and smashed

Knob fresh ginger, peeled and finely chopped

1 pinch red pepper flakes

¼ cup white wine vinegar

2/3 cup coconut aminos

2/3 cup beef stock

4 pounds beef ribs, chopped in half

2 tablespoons arrowroot

1-2 tablespoons water

DIRECTIONS (PREP + COOK TIME: 70 MINUTES)

Set your Ninja Foodi to Saute mode and add sesame oil, garlic, ginger, red pepper flakes and Saute for 1 minute. Deglaze pot with vinegar and mix in coconut aminos and beef stock Add ribs to the pot and coat them well. Lock lid and cook on HIGH pressure for 60 minutes Release pressure naturally over 10 minutes . Remove the ribs and keep them on the side Take a small bowl and mix in arrowroot and water, stir and mix in the liquid into the pot, set the pot to Saute mode and cook until the liquid reaches your desired consistency Put the ribs under a broiler to brown them slightly (also possible to do this in the Ninja Foodi using the Air Crisping lid) . Serve ribs with the cooking liquid. Enjoy!

Extremely Satisfying Beef Curry

INGREDIENTS (4 Servings)

2 pounds beef steak, cubed

2 tablespoons extra virgin olive oil

1 tablespoon Dijon mustard

2 and ½ tablespoons curry powder

2 yellow onions, peeled and chopped

2 garlic cloves, peeled and minced

10 ounces canned coconut milk

2 tablespoons tomato sauce

Salt and pepper to taste

DIRECTIONS (PREP + COOK TIME: 30 MINUTES)

Set your Ninja Foodi to "Saute" mode and add oil, let it heat up Add onions, garlic, stir cook for 4 minutes. Add mustard, stir and cook for 1 minute Add beef and stir until all sides are browned Add curry powder, salt, and pepper, stir cook for 2 minutes Add coconut milk and tomato sauce, stir, and cove Lock lid and cook on HIGH pressure for 10 minutes Release pressure naturally over 10 minutes. Serve and enjoy!

The Ground Beef Root Chili

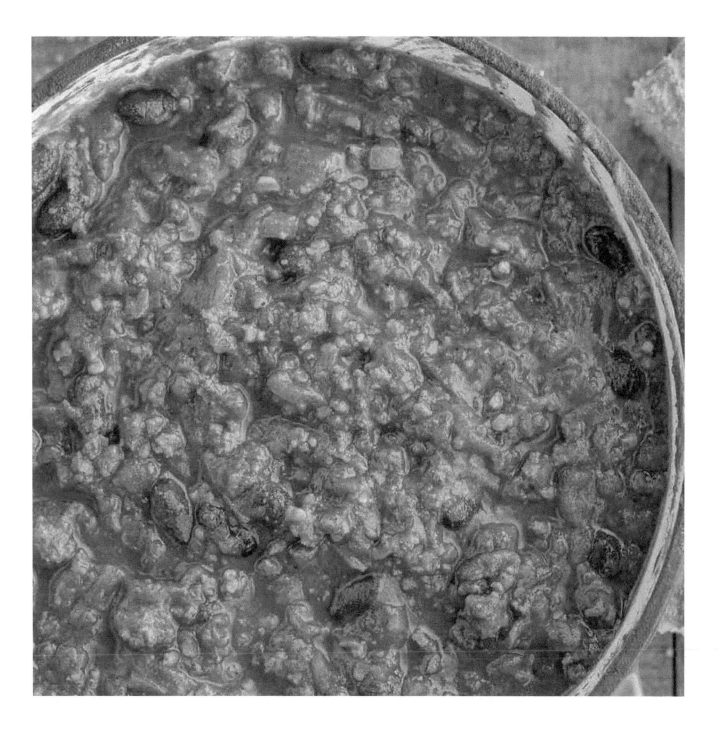

INGREDIENTS (6 Servings)

10 ounce of sliced beets

1 cup of cooked ground beef

1 and a 1/3 cup of diced carrot

1 and 1/3 cups of peeled and diced sweet potato

10 and a 2/3 ounce of pumpkin

1 teaspoon of dried rosemary

1 teaspoon of sea salt

2 teaspoon of dried basil

2/3 teaspoon of cinnamon

13 and a 1/3 of beef bone broth

1 and a 1/3 tablespoon of Apple Cider Vinegar

DIRECTIONS (PREP + COOK TIME: 25 MINUTES)

Add beets to a food processor and puree.Transfer the beets to your Ninja Foodi Add the rest of the ingredients . Lock up the lid and cook on HIGH pressure for 10 minutes Release the pressure naturally over 10 minutes. Enjoy!

Healthy Spinach Beef Prep

INGREDIENTS (4 Servings)

1 yellow onion; chopped

3 leeks, roughly chopped

2 tablespoons tomato puree

1 pound beef meat, ground

5 ounce baby spinach

1 tablespoon olive oil

Black pepper (finely ground) and salt to the taste

DIRECTIONS (Prep + Cook Time: 22-27 minutes) Take Ninja Foodi multi-cooker, arrange it over a cooking platform, and open the top lid. In the pot, add the oil; Select "SEAR/SAUTÉ" mode and select "MD: HI" pressure level. Press "STOP/START." After about 4-5 minutes, the oil will start simmering. Add the onions and cook (while stirring) until they become softened and translucent for 4-5 minutes. Add the leeks, stir, and cook for 2 minutes. Add the beef, salt, pepper, tomato puree, and the spinach; combine well. Seal the multi-cooker by locking it with the pressure lid; ensure to keep the pressure release valve locked/sealed. Select "PRESSURE" mode and select the "HI" pressure level. Then, set timer to 10 minutes and press "STOP/START"; it will start the cooking process by building up inside pressure. When the timer goes off, naturally release inside pressure for about 8-10 minutes. Then, quick-release pressure by adjusting the pressure valve to the VENT. Serve warm.

Barley Beef Stew

INGREDIENTS (5-6 Servings)

1 yellow onion; chopped

4 carrots; chopped

4 celery stalks; chopped

2 ½ pounds beef stew meat; cubed

15 ounce canned tomatoes; chopped

1 teaspoon oregano, dried

1 tablespoon olive oil

2 tablespoons tomato paste

6 cups beef stock

1 cup pearl barley

A pinch of black pepper (finely ground) and salt

DIRECTIONS (Prep + Cook Time: 40-45 minutes) Take Ninja Foodi multi-cooker, arrange it over a cooking platform, and open the top lid.   In the pot, add the oil; Select "SEAR/SAUTÉ" mode and select "MD: HI" pressure level. Press "STOP/START." After about 4-5 minutes, the oil will start simmering.   Add the beef and stir cook for about 5 minutes to brown evenly.   Add the onions, celery, carrots, oregano, salt and pepper, and cook (while stirring) until they become softened and translucent for 4-5 minutes.   Add the tomatoes, tomato paste, barley, and stock; stir gently.   Seal the multi-cooker by locking it with the pressure lid; ensure to keep the pressure release valve locked/sealed.   Select "PRESSURE" mode and select the "HI" pressure level. Then, set timer to 25 minutes and press "STOP/START"; it will start the cooking process by building up inside pressure.   When the timer goes off, naturally release inside pressure for about 8-10 minutes. Then, quick-release pressure by adjusting the pressure valve to the VENT.   Serve warm.

Moroccan Beef Mushroom Tagine

INGREDIENTS (6 Servings)

4 cups cremini mushrooms, sliced

2 pounds beef stew meat, cut in 2-inch cubes

2 tablespoons unsalted butter

1 yellow onion, diced

2 tablespoons soy sauce

2 cups chicken stock

2 teaspoons black pepper (ground)

2 sprigs thyme

2 tablespoons cornstarch

2 tablespoons water

1 (16-ounce) pack egg noodles

½ cup sour cream

DIRECTIONS (Prep + Cook Time: 23-28 minutes) Take Ninja Foodi multi-cooker, arrange it over a cooking platform, and open the top lid. In the pot, add the butter, Select "SEAR/SAUTÉ" mode and select "MD: HI" pressure level. Press "STOP/START." After about 4-5 minutes, the butter will melt. Add the onions, mushrooms, and cook (while stirring) until they become softened and translucent for 4-5 minutes. Add the beef, black pepper, thyme, soy sauce, and chicken stock. Simmer for 3 minutes. Seal the multi-cooker by locking it with the pressure lid, ensure to keep the pressure release valve locked/sealed. Select "PRESSURE" mode and select the "HI" pressure level. Then after, set timer to 10 minutes and press "STOP/START," it will start the cooking process by building up inside pressure. When the timer goes off, quickly release pressure by adjusting the pressure valve to the VENT. After pressure gets released, open the pressure lid. Add the egg noodles. Stir well. Seal the multi-cooker by locking it with the pressure lid, ensure to keep the pressure release valve locked/sealed. Select "PRESSURE" mode and select the "HI" pressure level. Then after, set timer to 5 minutes and press "STOP/START," it will start the cooking process by building up inside pressure. When the timer goes off, quickly release pressure by adjusting the pressure valve to the VENT. After pressure gets released, open the pressure lid. Combine the cornstarch and water until smooth. Add the mixture in the pot and stir well. Mix in the cream and serve warm.

Korean Chili Pork

INGREDIENTS (4 Servings)

2 pounds pork, cut into 1/8-inch slices

5 garlic cloves, minced

3 tablespoons green onion, minced

1 yellow onion, sliced

½ cup of soy sauce

½ cup brown sugar

3 tablespoons Korean Red Chili Paste

2 tablespoons sesame seeds

3 teaspoons black pepper

Red pepper flakes

DIRECTIONS (Prep + Cook Time: 13-18 minutes)

Take a zip bag and add listed ingredients, shake well and let it chill for 6-8 hours Pre-heat Ninja Foodi by pressing the "GRILL" option and setting it to "MED" and timer to 8 minutes Let it pre-heat until you hear a beep Arrange sliced pork over grill grate, lock lid and cook for 4 minutes Flip pork and cook for 4 minutes more, serve warm and enjoy with some chopped lettuce

Avocado Salsa Steak

INGREDIENTS (4 Servings)

1 cup cilantro leaves

2 ripe avocados, diced

2 cups salsa Verde

2 beef lank steak, diced

½ teaspoon salt

½ teaspoon pepper

2 medium tomatoes, seeded and diced

DIRECTIONS (Prep + Cook Time: 23-28 minutes) Rub beef steak with salt and pepper, season well Pre-heat Ninja Foodi by pressing the "GRILL" option and setting it to "MED" and timer to 18 minutes Let it pre-heat until you hear a beep Arrange diced steak over grill grate, lock lid and cook for 9 minutes Flip and cook for 9 minutes more Take a blender and blend in salsa, cilantro Serve with grilled steak, with blended salsa, tomato, and avocado Enjoy!

Herbed Beef Fillets

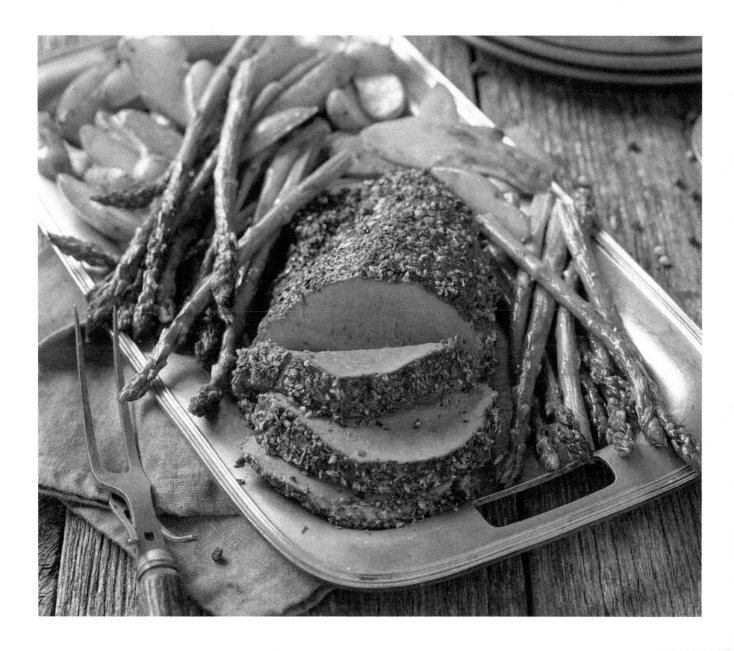

INGREDIENTS (2 Servings)

1 green bell pepper, cut into strips

½ tablespoon mustard

1 pound beef fillets, cut into strips

1 yellow onion, chopped

1 tablespoon olive oil

2 teaspoons Provencal herbs

Black pepper (ground) and salt to taste

DIRECTIONS (Prep + Cook Time: 20-25 minutes) Take Ninja Foodi multi-cooker, arrange it over a cooking platform, and open the top lid.　In the pot, add the oil, Select "SEAR/SAUTÉ" mode and select "MD: HI" pressure level. Press "STOP/START." After about 4-5 minutes, the oil will start simmering.　Add the onions, bell pepper, and cook (while stirring) until they become softened and translucent for 4-5 minutes.　Add the herbs, salt, black pepper, beef, and mustard, stir gently.　Seal the multi-cooker by locking it with the pressure lid, ensure to keep the pressure release valve locked/sealed.　Select "PRESSURE" mode and select the "HI" pressure level. Then after, set timer to 10 minutes and press "STOP/START," it will start the cooking process by building up inside pressure.   When the timer goes off, naturally release inside pressure for about 8-10 minutes. Then, quick-release pressure by adjusting the pressure valve to the VENT. Serve warm.

Beef Stroganoff with Egg Noodles

INGREDIENTS (6 Servings)

2 tablespoons of canola oil

1/2 onion, diced

2 teaspoons of salt, divided

2 pounds of beef stew meat, cut into cubes

1 teaspoon of ground black pepper

3 garlic cloves, diced finely

1/2 teaspoon of dried thyme

3 cups of mushrooms, chopped

2 tablespoons of soy sauce

2 tablespoons of all-purpose flour

3 glasses of chicken broth

1 (16 ounce) package of egg noodles

3/4 cup of sour cream

DIRECTIONS (PREP + COOK TIME: 57 MINUTES) Set your Foodi to sauté mode and add oil. Heat for a minute and add onions and a half teaspoon of salt. Stir. Cook for 3 to 4 minutes or until the onions begin to soften. Season the beef with a teaspoon of salt and pepper and add it to the Foodi. Cook for 2 minutes while stirring frequently until it browns evenly. Add thyme and garlic. Cook for around thirty seconds. Add soy sauce and mushrooms. Stir. Combine the Foodi content with flour. Add the chicken broth and the remaining salt. Close the pressure lid and cook on high mode for fifteen minutes. Quick release the pressure and open the lid.Add the egg noodles and close the crisping lid. Set the temperature to 360°F and set the Foodi to crisp mode for five minutes. When cooking is complete, open the Foodi and add the sour cream. Stir and serve.

Ragù Bolognese

INGREDIENTS (8 Servings)

1 cup of low-sodium chicken stock

4 packets (1 oz) of powdered gelatin

2 tablespoons of extra-virgin organic olive oil

1/2 lb of pancetta, finely diced

1 large onion (about 1 1/2 cups), minced finely

2 large carrots, chopped (about 1 cup)

2 large stalks of celery, chopped (about 1 cup)

4 medium garlic cloves, minced

1/4 cup of fresh sage leaves, minced

1/2 cup of parsley leaves, minced and divided

1/2 pound of chicken livers, minced

2 pounds of ground beef chuck

1 pound of ground pork shoulder

Kosher salt and freshly ground black pepper

1 (14-oz) can of crushed tomatoes

2 cups of dry red wine

1 1/2 cups of heavy cream, divided

2 bay leaves

3 oz of Parmesan cheese, finely grated

1 to 2 tablespoons of Thai fish sauce

1/4 cup of fresh basil leaves, minced

To Serve:

1 pound of dried penne, cooked

Finely grated Parmesan cheese

DIRECTIONS (PREP + COOK TIME: 110 MINUTES) Put the chicken stock in a bowl and sprinkle it with gelatin. Set aside. Sauté the pancetta in extra virgin olive oil for ten minutes or until browned. Add the onions, celery, carrots, sage, garlic, and half of the parsley. Cook the spices until they soften. Add the chicken livers and stir until the pinkness fades. Add beef, pork, salt, and pepper. Cook for 10 minutes or until the beef's redness fades while stirring frequently. Continue to cook-stir for around 25 minutes or until the excess fluid drains and the meat begins to sizzle. Add wine, the reserved mixture, tomatoes, a cup of heavy cream, and the bay leaves. Turn off the sauté function. Secure the pressure lid and cook the sautéed mixture on high mode for 35 minutes. Perform a quick release and open the lid. After that, simmer it on sauté mode to thicken. Add the remaining parsley, half cup of the heavy cream, fish sauce, and basil. Let it boil and season with salt and pepper. Serve your ragu Bolognese alongside the cooked pasta and parmesan.

Air Fried Beef Satay

INGREDIENTS (2 Servings)

1 lb of beef flank steak, sliced thinly

2 tablespoons of canola oil

1 tablespoon of fish sauce

A tablespoon of soy sauce

1 tablespoon of minced ginger,

A tablespoon of garlic, minced

1 teaspoon of Sriracha

A tablespoon of sugar

1 teaspoon of ground coriander

1/2 cup of chopped cilantro, divided

1/4 cup of roasted peanuts, chopped

DIRECTIONS (PREP + COOK TIME: 43 MINUTES) Get a Ziploc bag and stuff it with the beef strips, fish sauce, canola oil, ginger, garlic, cilantro(quarter cup,) coriander, Sriracha, soy sauce, and sugar. Toss. Marinate in the refrigerator for at least 30 minutes. Preheat the Foodi on Air Crisp Mode at 400°F. Insert the basket in the multi-cooker and transfer the beef-strip mixture in it (side by side.) Cook for 8 minutes at 400°F (flip once, halfway.) Ladle your air-fried beef into serving plates and top with the roasted peanuts and chopped cilantro.

Un-Stuffed Beef and Cabbage

INGREDIENTS (4 Servings)

2 lbs of organic beef

1 cabbage head, chopped

1 whole yellow onion

2 tablespoons of Italian seasoning

Salt and pepper

2 tablespoons of garlic, minced

1 14.5 oz of diced and canned tomatoes, juicy

1/2 cup of water

Shredded cheese

DIRECTIONS (PREP + COOK TIME: 25 MINUTES) Set the Foodi unit to sear/sauté mode over medium-high temperatures. Add the beef and brown it while breaking up large lumps.   Add the onions, seasoning, garlic, pepper, and salt. Cook while stirring for 5 minutes and turn off the sauté mode.   Add the chopped cabbage to the beef mixture. Add the canned tomatoes. Secure the pressure lid and cook on high mode for 5 minutes.   Quick release the pressure and open the lid.   Add the shredded cheese and close the crisping lid. Air-fry it for 3 minutes at a temperature of 390°F.

Balsamic Roast Beef

INGREDIENTS (6 Servings)

1 (3 lb.) of boneless roast beef

1 cup of beef broth

1 tablespoon of Worcestershire sauce

1/2 cup of balsamic vinegar

1 tablespoon of honey

A tablespoon of soy sauce

1/2 teaspoon of red pepper flakes

4 garlic cloves, chopped

DIRECTIONS (PREP + COOK TIME: 50 MINUTES) Put the roast beef in the Foodi. Combine the beef broth with Worcestershire sauce, balsamic vinegar, soy sauce, red pepper flakes, honey, and garlic in a bowl. Secure the pressure lid and cook on high mode for 30 minutes. Release the pressure naturally for 15 minutes and open the lid. Remove the roast from the pot but reserve its gravy. Serve your balsamic roast meat alongside its gravy.

Air fryer Lamb Chops

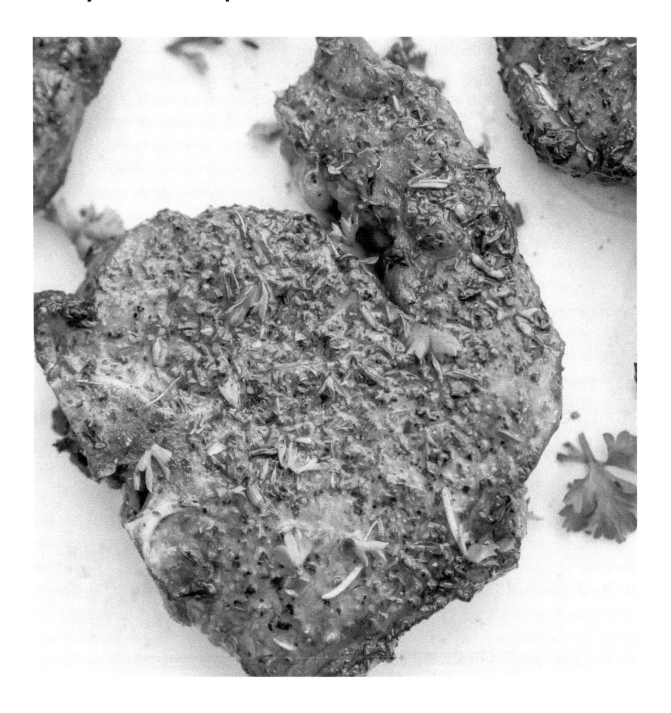

INGREDIENTS (2 Servings)

4 lamb chops

2 tablespoons of canola oil Garlic herb

1/2 tablespoons of finely chopped fresh oregano

1 garlic cloves   Kosher salt

DIRECTIONS (PREP + COOK TIME: 20 MINUTES) Preheat the Foodi unit on bake/roast at 350°F.   Coat the garlic clove with a half teaspoon of oil and place it in the crisping basket. Meanwhile, combine the oregano with half teaspoon of canola oil, salt, and pepper. Coat the lamb chops with the oregano mixture and leave it for 2-3 minutes. Once the garlic bulb browns, remove it and preheat the unit on air crisp mode at 390°F. Put the lamb chops into the basket and set it to 350°F. Air-fry the chops for 5-10 minutes or until they brown. Transfer to a dish. Squeeze the garlic cloves into the remaining oil. Add salt and pepper. Stir well and serve the lamp chops with the garlic sauce.

Steak, Potatoes and Asparagus

INGREDIENTS (4 Servings)

5 Russet potatoes (peeled and cut in ½" pieces)

1/2 cup of water

1/2 cup of heavy cream

1/4 cup of butter, divided

1 cup of cheddar cheese, shredded

3 teaspoons of ground black pepper, divided

1 tablespoon plus

2 teaspoons of kosher salt, divided

2 frozen New York strip steaks (12 oz. each, 1 1/2 inches thick)

1 trimmed asparagus

1 tablespoon of organic olive oil

DIRECTIONS (PREP + COOK TIME: 20 MINUTES) Add potatoes and water to the Foodi. Insert the reversible rack in the pot and add the frozen steak (previously seasoned salt and pepper.) Secure the pressure lid and cook the steak strips on high mode for a minute. Add asparagus, oil, a teaspoon of salt, and pepper. Cook the asparagus on high mode for another minute. Quick release the accumulated vapor and open the lid. Remove the rack and transfer the steaks to a bowl. Pat-dry them. Mash the potatoes and add a quarter cup of butter, cheese, cream, a teaspoon of salt, and pepper. Return the dry steak to the Foodi and insert a rack containing asparagus into it. Close the crisping lid and cook on broil mode for 8-12 minutes. Leave the steak to dry for around five minutes and serve it alongside the mashed potatoes and baked asparagus.

Keto Chunky Chili

INGREDIENTS (6 Servings)

1¼ lbs of ground beef

1 tablespoon of essential olive oil

½ mid-sized yellow onion, chopped

2 garlic cloves, peeled and minced

2 teaspoons of cumin

1½ tablespoons of chili powder

1½ teaspoons of sea salt

1 teaspoons of garlic powder

A teaspoon of smoked paprika

¼ teaspoon of coriander powder

1/8 teaspoon of red pepper cayenne

1 cup of beef broth

2/3 cup of water

¼ cup of canned pumpkin (unsweetened)

1 cup of canned diced tomatoes

2 tablespoons of tomato paste

1 cup of zucchini squash, diced

2/3 cup of cauliflower, finely chopped

Optional toppings:

2/3 cup of grated cheddar cheese,

½ avocado, chopped

3 tablespoons of sour cream, optional

DIRECTIONS (PREP + COOK TIME: 45 MINUTES) Set the Foodi to sauté mode. Preheat it for a minute and then add the organic olive oil and ground beef. Sauté for 5minutes while splitting up the beef using a wooden spoon. After browning the beef, add the chopped onions and the minced garlic. Sauté until the garlic becomes translucent. Add the remaining ingredients (except the toppings) and stir. Close the pressure lid and cook them on high mode for 25 minutes. Allow the pressure to exit naturally for 10 minutes and quick release the rest. Open the lid and stir. Serve your Keto chunky chilli with the toppings.

Beef and Egg Noodles

INGREDIENTS (4 Servings)

3 lbs of beef chuck roast, cubed

2- 3 cups of water

4 cups of beef stock

1 1/2 lbs of Crimini mushrooms, quartered

1 medium onion (sliced and quartered)

A dry onion soup mix

2 tablespoons of sunflower oil

2 garlic cloves, minced

2 tablespoons of soy sauce

1 teaspoon of marjoram, dried

A teaspoon of Worcestershire sauce

1 teaspoon of garlic powder

1 teaspoon of onion powder

1/2 teaspoon of thyme

A tablespoon of kitchen bouquet (optional)

1/4 cup of flour

Salt and pepper

DIRECTIONS (PREP + COOK TIME: 60 MINUTES) Sauté the beef cubes in sunflower oil for 15 minutes or until they brown. Stir and add onions, spices, garlic, and the onion soup mix. Add the mushrooms, Worcestershire, soy, and stock. Stir. Add some water and lock the pressure lid. Cook the mixture on high mode for 45 minutes. Release the pressure naturally and open the lid. Add flour and the kitchen browning sauce to thicken the gravy. Add salt and pepper, if required. Serve your beef meal alongside egg noodles.

Keto Curried Beef

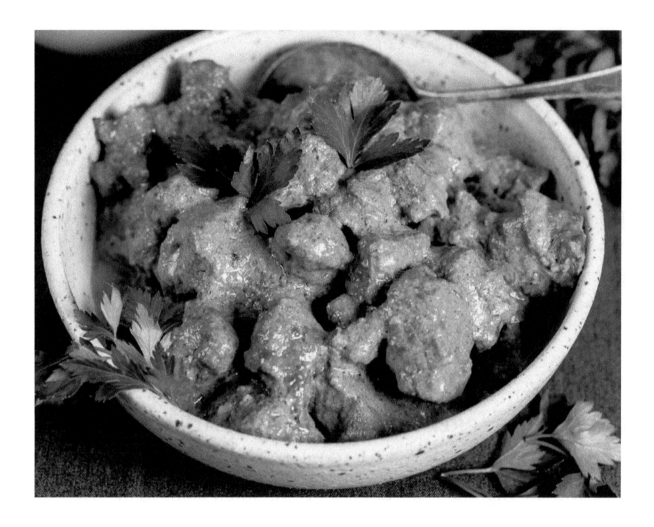

INGREDIENTS (4 Servings)

1 tablespoon of coconut oil

1.5 lbs of stew beef meat

1/2 medium white onion, diced

2 teaspoons of curry powder

3 teaspoons of minced garlic

1 teaspoon of cumin

1/2 teaspoon of chili powder

A teaspoon of Pink Himalayan

Salt 1 can of coconut milk, refrigerated

1/2 cup of Water

DIRECTIONS (PREP + COOK TIME: 40 MINUTES) Put the coconut milk in the freezer for at least one hour. Set your Foodi to sear/sauté mode and add a half tablespoon of coconut oil. Add the beef and brown it lightly. Add the remaining coconut oil and the diced onion. Cook until the onions become translucent. Add garlic, cumin, curry powder, and chili powder. Stir and cook until they fragrant. Return the stew meat in the Foodi and add some water. Close the pressure lid and cook the beef mixture on high mode for ten minutes. Quick release the accumulated vapor and open the lid. Remove the coconut milk from the freezer and discard the floating liquid. Add the hardened coconut milk to the beef mixture and stir. Simmer the mixture on sauté mode for 10 minutes or until the milk melts and the curry sauce thicken. Enjoy!

Tex-Mex Meatloaf

INGREDIENTS (6 Servings)

1 pound of uncooked ground beef

1 bell pepper, diced

1 egg

1/2 jalapeño pepper (deseeded and minced)

1 small onion (peeled and diced)

3 corn tortillas, chopped roughly

1 tablespoon of garlic powder

2 teaspoons of chili powder

2 teaspoons of ground cumin

1 teaspoon of cayenne pepper

2 teaspoons of kosher salt

Barbecue sauce

1/4 cup of fresh cilantro leaves

A cup of water

1 cup of corn chips, crushed

DIRECTIONS (PREP + COOK TIME: 30 MINUTES) Combine all the ingredients (except the corn cheese and barbecue sauce) in a bowl. Transfer the mixture into a loaf pan of 8 ½" and cover with foil. Pour water in the pot. Put the pan on a reversible rack and fix the rack in the Foodi. Lock the pressure lid and cook the mixture on high mode for 15 minutes. Quick release the accumulated vapor and open the lid. Remove the foil and close the crisping lid. Set your pot to bake/roast mode, temperature to 360°F, and timer to 15 minutes. Meanwhile, mix two tablespoons of barbecue sauce with corn chips in a bowl. Add the barbecue mixture to the pot on the eighth minute and close the lid. Let the mixture cook to completion. Transfer the meat loaf to a serving bowl and enjoy.

Beef Gyros

Peppercinis Pot Roast

INGREDIENTS (4-6 Servings)

(1) 3-4 lb roast   1 packet of ranch seasoning mix

1 stick (1/2 cup) of butter

½ jar of Peppercinis, juice inclusive

½ cup of water

DIRECTIONS (PREP + COOK TIME: 105 MINUTES) Put the roast in the Foodi and sprinkle the ranch mix over it.   Add butter, peppercinis, and water.   Secure the pressure lid and cook on high mode for 90 minutes. Quick release the in-built pressure and open the lid carefully. Shred your pot roast and serve!

Dinner of Beef Short Ribs Appetizing!

INGREDIENTS (4 Servings)

1 teaspoon of onion salt

A teaspoon of rosemary

1/2 teaspoon of paprika

1/2 teaspoon of sage

1/2 teaspoon of ground pepper

2 lbs of beef short rib

2 tablespoons of oil

1 (6oz) can of tomato paste

1/2 cup of balsamic vinegar

1/2 cup of water

2 tablespoons of Dijon mustard

1 tablespoon of hot chocolate mix, unsweetened

6 cloves garlic

DIRECTIONS (PREP + COOK TIME: 50 MINUTES)

Combine sage with rosemary, pepper, paprika, and onion salt in a bowl. Rub the beef short ribs with the mixture. Sauté the ribs with oil and set aside. Add water, tomato paste, balsamic, cocoa, Dijon mustard, and garlic in the Foodi and mix. Add the seasoned short ribs. Secure the pressure lid and cook on high mode for 40 minutes. Quick release the in-built pressure and open the lid. Ladle sauce over the beef ribs and enjoy!

Shredded Beef Sloppy Joes

INGREDIENTS (10 Servings)

6 lbs of boneless chuck, cubed

1/2 cup of red chili sauce

1 tablespoon of garlic, minced

1/2 cup of water

2 tablespoons of olive oil

1 cup of barbecue sauce

1 onion, chopped

DIRECTIONS (PREP + COOK TIME: 70 MINUTES) Put some oil in the Foodi and add the minced garlic. Sauté the garlic for 30 seconds. Brown the meat and add the barbeque sauce, red chili sauce, onion, and water. Close the pressure lid and cook on high mode for 50 minutes. Quick release the in-built pressure and open the lid. Transfer the beef to a cutting board and shred. Return it and add more barbeque sauce. Serve alongside buns.

Beef and Old-School Calico Beans

INGREDIENTS (8 Servings)

A pound of ground beef

1 pound of bacon or bacon pieces

1 large can of pork and beans

1 large onion, chopped

2 cans (15 ½-oz) of kidney beans, drained

2 cans (15 ½- oz) of butter beans, drained

3 cups of stewed tomatoes

½ cup of sugar 1 cup of corn

¾ cup of brown sugar

½ cup of ketchup

1 teaspoon of mustard

3 tablespoons of cider vinegar

A teaspoon of garlic, ground

1 tablespoon of water(for smoking)

DIRECTIONS (PREP + COOK TIME: 45 MINUTES) Brown the bacon on sauté mode. Break it down to form drippings. Add the hamburger and onions. Brown them until all the fats drains. Combine all the ingredients (including the drippings) in the Foodi and pressure cook for 25 minutes. Enjoy.

Beef Short Ribs and Vegetables

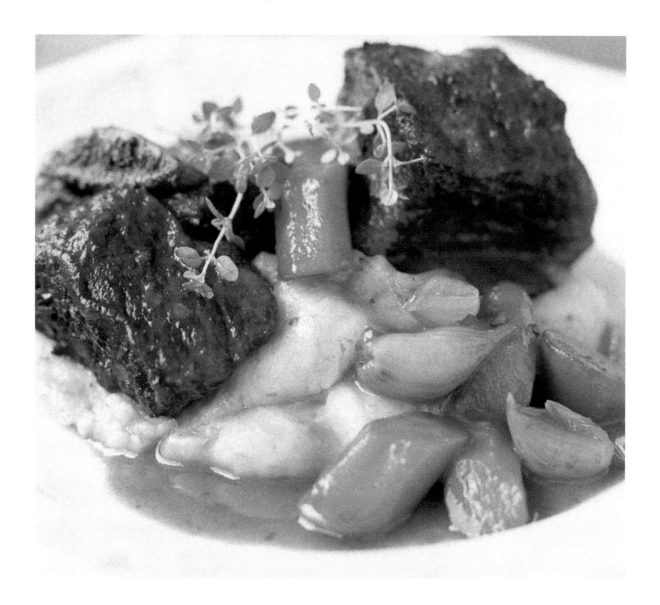

INGREDIENTS (4 -6Servings)

6 uncooked beef short ribs (about 3 lb), bony but trimmed

2 teaspoons of black pepper, divided

2 teaspoons of kosher salt, divided

2 tablespoons of olive oil, divided

1 onion (peeled and chopped)

1/4 cup of beef broth

1/4 cup of Masala wine

2 tablespoons of brown sugar

2 tablespoons of fresh thyme, (minced and divided)

3 cloves garlic, (peeled and minced)

3 carrots (peeled and cut into 1" pieces)

3 parsnips (peeled and cut into 1" pieces)

1 cup of pearl onions

1/4 cup of fresh minced parsley

DIRECTIONS (PREP + COOK TIME: 75 MINUTES) Begin by seasoning the short ribs with a teaspoon of salt and pepper. Allow it to sauté for 10 minutes or until both sides turns brown. Add wine, onion, broth, garlic, brown sugar, a tablespoon of thyme, a half teaspoon of salt, and pepper. Secure the pressure lid and cook the mixture on high mode for 40 minutes. Halfway, open the lid and add carrots, pearl onions, parsnips, the remaining thyme, oil, salt, and pepper. After pressure cooking, quick release the accumulated steam and open the lid. Insert the crisping rack and put the vegetables in it. Close the crisping lid and bake at 350°F for fifteen minutes. After that, transfer the baked veggies and ribs to a tray and cover to keep warm. Sauté the remaining liquid for 5 minutes and pour it into another bowl. Spoon off the fatty layer and add the parsley. Stir. Serve your short ribs and veggies alongside the prepared sauce.

Conclusion

Did you appreciate trying these new and also delicious recipes?>

Unfortunately we have actually come to the end of this cookbook regarding using the great Ninja Foodi multi-cooker, which I truly hope you delighted in.>

To boost your health we want to recommend you to combine physical activity and also a vibrant way of life along with following these wonderful dishes, so regarding highlight the improvements. we will certainly be back soon with an increasing number of intriguing vegetarian recipes, a huge hug, see you soon.

CPSIA information can be obtained
at www.ICGtesting.com
Printed in the USA
LVHW102315220621
690925LV00016B/1415